I Hate My Body

Embracing the Beauty Within and a Journey to Self-Love

Within These Pages Lies a Beacon of Light

Note from the author.

In a world that bombards us with impossible beauty standards and fosters a culture of comparison, many individuals find themselves trapped in a relentless cycle of body self-loathing. The weight of societal pressures and negative self-perceptions can cast a shadow over our lives, hindering our happiness and preventing us from fully embracing the beauty within us.

But amidst this sea of self-doubt, there is hope. Within these pages lies a beacon of light, a guidebook that will help you navigate the depths of body self-loathing and emerge victorious on the path to self-love. "Embracing the Beauty Within: A Journey to Self-Love" is not just another book; it is a transformative companion designed to empower and uplift you.

This book is a testament to the strength and resilience of the human spirit. It draws upon years of research, personal experiences, and the wisdom of experts who have dedicated their lives to understanding the intricacies of body image and self-worth. It offers you a sanctuary where you can find solace, guidance, and practical tools to navigate the treacherous terrain of body self-loathing.

Within these pages, you will embark on a profound journey of self-discovery. You will uncover the underlying causes of your body self-loathing, delving into the societal influences, media messages, and personal experiences that have shaped your perception of beauty. As you explore the psychological and emotional factors at play, you will gain invaluable insights into your own unique struggles.

But this book does not stop at the analysis of the problem. It goes beyond, providing you with real answers and tangible solutions. You will encounter strategies to challenge societal norms, embrace body diversity, and foster self-acceptance. Practical exercises and transformative practices will guide you towards cultivating self-compassion, nurturing your self-esteem, and redefining your relationship with your body.

The wisdom contained within these pages is not meant to be passively absorbed; it is meant to be put into action. It is an invitation to embrace your own power, to take charge of your thoughts, beliefs, and actions. It empowers you to reclaim your self-worth, to rewrite the narrative of your body story, and to embark on a lifelong journey towards self-love.

As you embark on this transformative journey, remember that you are not alone.

Countless others have walked a similar path, fighting their way out of the darkness and into the radiant embrace of self-acceptance. Their stories, shared within this book, will inspire you, uplift you, and remind you that you are worthy of love, respect, and happiness.

Dear reader, within these pages, you hold the key to unlock the door to your own liberation. As you embark on this journey, be gentle with yourself, for healing takes time. Embrace the beauty within you, for it is vast and boundless. Let the insights, answers, and solutions contained in this book guide you towards a future filled with self-love, confidence, and an unwavering appreciation for the extraordinary person you truly are.

With love and unwavering support,

Phoenix Bloom

Chapters

Chapter 1:
Understanding Body Dissatisfaction

Defining body dissatisfaction and its impact on mental and emotional well-being.

Examining the societal and cultural factors that contribute to body dissatisfaction.

Exploring the psychological and emotional aspects underlying body dissatisfaction.

Chapter 2:
Unraveling Beauty Standards

Analyzing the influence of media, advertising, and social platforms on beauty ideals.

Discussing the impact of unrealistic beauty standards on body image.

Challenging societal norms and promoting body diversity and inclusivity.

Chapter 3:
The Psychology of Body Image

Exploring the psychological factors contributing to body dissatisfaction.

Discussing the role of self-esteem, self-worth, and identity in body image.

Examining the relationship between body image and mental health.

Chapter 4:
Developing a Healthy Body Image

Promoting self-acceptance and positive body image.

Encouraging self-compassion and self-care practices.

Providing strategies to improve body confidence and self-esteem.

Chapter 5:
Navigating Social Pressures

Addressing the impact of social comparison and peer pressure on body image.

Discussing strategies for handling societal pressures and negative comments.

Promoting assertiveness and setting healthy boundaries.

Chapter 6:
Cultivating Self-Care Practices

Encouraging holistic well-being beyond physical appearance.

Exploring self-care practices that promote body and mind nourishment.

Discussing the importance of self-compassion, mindfulness, and stress management.

Chapter 7:
Building a Supportive Environment

Highlighting the role of relationships and social support in body image.

Offering advice on fostering positive relationships and supportive communities.

Discussing how to address body image concerns within families, friendships, and romantic partnerships.

Chapter 8:
Seeking Professional Help

Recognizing when body dissatisfaction becomes severe and impacts mental health.

Providing information on seeking professional assistance, such as therapists or counselors.

Exploring evidence-based interventions and therapies for body image concerns.

Chapter 9:
Embracing Body Positivity and Activism

Discussing the body positivity movement and its impact on self-acceptance.

Encouraging readers to participate in body positivity activism.

Exploring ways to challenge societal beauty norms and promote inclusivity.

Chapter 10:
Sustaining Body Acceptance for the Long Term

Providing strategies for maintaining a positive body image in the face of challenges.

Addressing setbacks and relapses in body acceptance.

Offering guidance on embracing body acceptance as a lifelong journey.

Chapter 1

Defining body dissatisfaction and its impact on mental and emotional well-being.

1. Understanding Body Dissatisfaction:
  - Define body dissatisfaction as the negative evaluation or dissatisfaction with one's body shape, size, weight, or specific body parts.
  - Explain that body dissatisfaction often involves a discrepancy between one's perceived body image and societal beauty standards.
  - Highlight that body dissatisfaction can affect individuals of any gender, age, or body size.

2. The Emotional Toll of Body Dissatisfaction:
  - Explore the emotional consequences of body dissatisfaction, such as low self-esteem, self-worth, and self-confidence.
  - Discuss the impact of body dissatisfaction on mood, including increased risk of depression, anxiety, and disordered eating behaviors.
  - Explain how negative body image can lead to social withdrawal, isolation, and diminished quality of life.

3. Body Dissatisfaction and Mental Health:

- Examine the link between body dissatisfaction and various mental health conditions, such as body dysmorphic disorder (BDD), eating disorders, and depression.
- Discuss the potential development of maladaptive coping strategies, such as excessive exercise, restrictive dieting, or engaging in unhealthy behaviors to attain an idealized body image.
- Highlight the vicious cycle between body dissatisfaction and negative mental health outcomes.

4. Societal Influences on Body Dissatisfaction:
- Explore how societal factors, including media, advertising, and social media, perpetuate unrealistic beauty ideals that contribute to body dissatisfaction.
- Discuss the impact of objectification, body shaming, and appearance-focused messages on individuals' perceptions of their bodies.
- Examine the role of cultural and societal norms in shaping body ideals and the subsequent impact on body dissatisfaction.

5. Intersectionality and Body Dissatisfaction:
- Recognize that experiences of body dissatisfaction can be influenced by intersectional

factors such as race, ethnicity, sexual orientation, and disability.
   - Discuss how marginalized groups may face unique challenges and pressures related to body image.
   - Highlight the importance of acknowledging and addressing the intersectional aspects of body dissatisfaction.

6. The Need for Body Acceptance and Positive Body Image:
   - Emphasize the importance of promoting body acceptance and a positive body image as essential components of mental and emotional well-being.
   - Discuss research and evidence that supports the connection between body acceptance and improved psychological outcomes.
   - Introduce concepts such as body neutrality, self-compassion, and appreciating body functionality beyond appearance.

By exploring these aspects, readers can gain a comprehensive understanding of body dissatisfaction and its impact on mental and emotional well-being. Providing relevant research findings, case studies, and personal stories can further enhance the chapter's effectiveness in conveying the significance of addressing body dissatisfaction for overall well-being.

Examining the societal and cultural factors that contribute to body dissatisfaction.

Examining the societal and cultural factors that contribute to body dissatisfaction sheds light on the complex web of influences that shape our perceptions of beauty and body image. Here's an explanation of these factors:

1. Media Influence: Media plays a significant role in shaping beauty ideals and perpetuating body dissatisfaction. Advertising, movies, television shows, magazines, and social media often showcase highly edited and unrealistic images of bodies. These images create an unattainable standard of beauty, leading individuals to compare themselves unfavorably and feel dissatisfied with their own bodies.

2. Beauty Standards: Societal beauty standards are deeply ingrained in cultural norms and values. These standards vary across cultures and time periods but often prioritize certain body types, features, or physical characteristics. The pressure to conform to these standards can lead to body dissatisfaction, as individuals may feel inadequate or unworthy if they do not meet the prescribed ideals.

3. Objectification and Sexualization: Society's tendency to objectify and sexualize bodies can contribute to body dissatisfaction. When bodies are reduced to mere objects of desire or judged solely on their appearance, individuals may feel reduced to their physical attributes and constantly evaluate themselves based on external judgments.

4. Social Comparison: Humans have a natural inclination to compare themselves to others, and social comparison is amplified in today's interconnected world. Constant exposure to carefully curated images on social media platforms fuels the tendency to compare one's body to those of others, leading to negative self-perceptions and body dissatisfaction.

5. Family and Peer Influence: Family and peer environments can significantly impact body image. Negative comments, criticisms, or pressures from family members or peers can shape an individual's perception of their own body. In particular, comments about weight, appearance, or body shape can be particularly influential and contribute to body dissatisfaction.

6. Cultural Factors: Cultural beliefs and practices surrounding beauty, body size, and shape can

strongly influence body image. Some cultures may idealize specific body types or emphasize the importance of appearance, leading individuals to internalize these cultural expectations and experience body dissatisfaction if they do not align with the ideal.

7. Historical and Societal Changes: Beauty ideals and body preferences have evolved throughout history and vary across societies. Changes in fashion trends, beauty standards, and societal norms contribute to shifting expectations and can create pressure to conform to new ideals. These changes can exacerbate body dissatisfaction as individuals strive to meet ever-changing standards.

Examining these societal and cultural factors that contribute to body dissatisfaction is essential for understanding the complex nature of the problem. By recognizing and challenging these influences, we can work towards creating a more inclusive and body-positive society. Promoting media literacy, embracing diverse beauty standards, challenging objectification, fostering positive family and peer environments, and promoting self-acceptance are crucial steps towards reducing body dissatisfaction and promoting a healthier body image.

Meet Sarah. She's a vibrant young woman with a zest for life, but lately, she's been feeling down. Sarah often finds herself standing in front of the mirror, scrutinizing every inch of her body. She sees flaws where others see beauty, and this self-criticism has taken a toll on her mental and emotional well-being.

Body dissatisfaction refers to the negative evaluation or dissatisfaction individuals experience with their bodies. It's like wearing tinted glasses that blur their perception of themselves. For Sarah, it means focusing on perceived imperfections and comparing herself to unrealistic beauty standards set by the media and society.

The impact of body dissatisfaction on Sarah's mental and emotional well-being has been significant. She often experiences low self-esteem, feeling unworthy and unattractive. It's as if her confidence has been chipped away, affecting her interactions with others and how she perceives herself in social situations.

Sarah's negative body image has also taken a toll on her emotional state. She often feels anxious and self-conscious, constantly worrying about how others perceive her. These feelings can escalate into symptoms of depression, as the weight of her dissatisfaction begins to overshadow her everyday experiences and joys.

But Sarah's story is not unique. Body dissatisfaction can affect anyone, regardless of their gender, age, or body size. It permeates through society, fueled by media, advertising, and social media platforms that bombard us with airbrushed and digitally manipulated images. These images create unrealistic ideals that few can attain, leading to a constant sense of falling short.

The consequences of body dissatisfaction extend beyond surface-level concerns. It seeps into the depths of mental health, impacting individuals' overall well-being. Studies have shown that body dissatisfaction increases the risk of developing eating disorders, such as anorexia or bulimia, as individuals resort to extreme measures in pursuit of an idealized body shape or weight.

The psychological distress caused by body dissatisfaction can also contribute to the development or exacerbation of conditions like body dysmorphic disorder (BDD), a mental health disorder characterized by an obsessive preoccupation with perceived flaws in one's appearance. In the case of BDD, the dissatisfaction with one's body becomes all-consuming, affecting daily functioning and overall quality of life.

Moreover, body dissatisfaction can create a vicious cycle. The negative emotions associated with a poor body image lead individuals to engage in maladaptive coping strategies. For some, this might involve excessive exercise, extreme dieting, or even turning to harmful substances. These behaviors can further damage mental and emotional well-being, perpetuating the cycle of dissatisfaction and despair.

It is crucial to understand the societal influences that shape body dissatisfaction. Media, advertising, and social media platforms play a significant role in perpetuating unrealistic beauty standards. They bombard us with images that have been meticulously edited, presenting an unattainable and narrow version of beauty. This constant exposure to idealized bodies can warp our perceptions and make us feel inadequate.

Recognizing and addressing body dissatisfaction requires a holistic approach. It involves fostering a positive body image, promoting self-acceptance, and challenging societal norms. It's about understanding that beauty comes in all shapes, sizes, and forms. By cultivating self-compassion, embracing body functionality, and nurturing a supportive environment, individuals like Sarah can begin their journey toward healing and self-love.

This narrative sets the stage for the chapter, introducing Sarah as a relatable character and highlighting the impact of body dissatisfaction on her mental and emotional well-being. It emphasizes the connection between body image and overall well-being, paving the way for further exploration and discussion in the subsequent sections of the chapter.

Exploring the psychological and emotional aspects underlying body dissatisfaction.

Body dissatisfaction is not solely a superficial issue but has deep psychological and emotional roots that contribute to its development and persistence. Understanding these underlying aspects is crucial in addressing body dissatisfaction effectively.

1. Self-Esteem and Self-Worth: Body dissatisfaction often stems from low self-esteem and a diminished sense of self-worth. Individuals may tie their value and worthiness to their physical appearance, leading to self-criticism and

negative evaluations when they perceive their bodies as falling short of societal ideals.

2. Social Comparison: Humans have a natural tendency to compare themselves to others, particularly in terms of appearance. In the age of social media, constant exposure to carefully curated images of others can intensify this social comparison. Individuals may compare their bodies to the seemingly "perfect" bodies of others, which can fuel feelings of inadequacy and dissatisfaction.

3. Perfectionism: Body dissatisfaction often intersects with perfectionism. Individuals may strive for an unrealistic and unattainable ideal of physical perfection. The pursuit of this ideal can result in relentless self-criticism, setting unreasonably high standards, and experiencing chronic dissatisfaction with one's body.

4. Internalization of Societal Ideals: The internalization of societal beauty standards plays a significant role in body dissatisfaction. Individuals may absorb and adopt these ideals as their own, striving to conform to an unrealistic physical ideal. This internalization can distort their perception of their bodies and contribute to negative body image.

5. Media Influence: Media, including advertising, movies, and magazines, heavily influence body dissatisfaction. The portrayal of thin, flawless, and highly edited bodies as the beauty ideal creates an unattainable standard. Exposure to these images can shape individuals' beliefs about their own bodies, perpetuating dissatisfaction and negative self-perception.

6. Objectification: Body dissatisfaction is often intertwined with the objectification of the body. When individuals perceive their bodies solely as objects to be evaluated and judged based on appearance, it can fuel dissatisfaction and lead to self-objectification. This perspective can diminish their overall well-being and contribute to negative body image.

Understanding the psychological and emotional aspects underlying body dissatisfaction provides insight into the complexity of this issue. By addressing these underlying factors, interventions and strategies can be developed to promote a healthier body image and improve overall well-being.

In conclusion, body dissatisfaction is influenced by a range of psychological and emotional aspects. Low self-esteem, social comparison, perfectionism, internalization of societal ideals, media influence, and objectification all contribute to the development and perpetuation of body dissatisfaction. Recognizing and addressing these underlying factors is essential in promoting body acceptance, fostering positive self-perception, and improving individuals' psychological and emotional well-being. By cultivating self-compassion, promoting realistic ideals, and challenging societal beauty norms, we can create a more inclusive and body-positive culture that supports individuals in developing a healthier relationship with their bodies.

Chapter2

Analyzing the influence of media, advertising, and social platforms on beauty ideals

Media, advertising, and social platforms play a significant role in shaping beauty ideals and have a profound impact on body dissatisfaction. Analyzing their influence helps us understand how these forces contribute to unrealistic standards and promote body dissatisfaction.

1. Unrealistic Portrayals: Media, such as magazines, movies, and television, often present an idealized and narrow version of beauty. Photoshopped images, airbrushing, and digitally manipulated bodies create an unrealistic and unattainable standard. This constant exposure to flawless and perfected bodies can distort perceptions, leading individuals to compare themselves unfavorably and feel dissatisfied with their own appearance.

2. Advertising and Commercialization: Advertisements heavily capitalize on insecurities to sell products. They often perpetuate the idea that one's body needs improvement or that there

is a flaw to be fixed. By associating beauty and desirability with certain products, they create a culture of dissatisfaction and the belief that one's worth is linked to external appearance.

3. Social Media Influence: Social platforms amplify the impact of media and advertising on body dissatisfaction. Users often curate and showcase their lives, including their appearance, creating a constant stream of seemingly perfect bodies. The pressure to conform to these carefully crafted images can lead to increased self-comparison and dissatisfaction. Moreover, social media platforms provide a breeding ground for appearance-focused judgments, cyberbullying, and body-shaming, further exacerbating body dissatisfaction.

4. Lack of Diversity: Media and advertising historically have had a limited representation of diverse body types, shapes, sizes, and ethnicities. This lack of diversity reinforces narrow beauty ideals, excluding individuals who do not fit within those standards. The underrepresentation of diverse bodies can perpetuate feelings of exclusion and inadequacy among those who do not conform to the predominant beauty ideals.

5. Reinforcement of Beauty Stereotypes: Media, advertising, and social platforms often perpetuate harmful stereotypes regarding beauty, such as associating thinness with worth or equating attractiveness with specific features. These stereotypes limit the appreciation and celebration of diverse beauty and contribute to the internalization of unrealistic and harmful beauty standards.

In conclusion, media, advertising, and social platforms significantly influence beauty ideals and have a substantial impact on body dissatisfaction. Unrealistic portrayals, commercialization of insecurities, social media pressures, lack of diversity, and the reinforcement of beauty stereotypes all contribute to the perpetuation of unattainable beauty standards. Recognizing and challenging these influences is essential in promoting body acceptance, fostering diversity and inclusivity, and nurturing positive body image. By advocating for more authentic representations and promoting media literacy, we can help individuals develop a healthier relationship with their bodies and challenge the harmful effects of media and advertising on beauty ideals.

Discussing the impact of unrealistic beauty standards on body image.

Unrealistic beauty standards imposed by society have a profound impact on body image, contributing to body dissatisfaction and negative self-perception. Understanding this impact sheds light on the detrimental consequences and highlights the need for promoting a more realistic and inclusive definition of beauty.

1. Internalizing Unattainable Ideals: Unrealistic beauty standards often portray an idealized body image that is virtually unattainable for the majority of individuals. These standards emphasize specific body shapes, sizes, and features, creating an unrelenting pressure to conform. Internalizing these ideals leads to constant self-comparison and dissatisfaction, as individuals perceive their bodies as falling short of the perceived norm.

2. Distorted Body Perception: Exposure to unrealistic beauty standards can distort individuals' perception of their own bodies. They may develop a skewed perception of what is considered normal or desirable. This distortion can lead to body dysmorphia, a condition characterized by an obsessive focus on perceived flaws in one's appearance, even when they may not objectively exist.

3. Negative Body Image: Unrealistic beauty standards foster negative body image, causing individuals to view their bodies negatively and fixate on perceived imperfections. They may engage in body-shaming self-talk, constantly criticizing and devaluing their physical appearance. This negative body image can erode self-esteem, self-confidence, and overall well-being.

4. Impact on Mental Health: The relentless pursuit of unattainable beauty standards can have significant implications for mental health. It contributes to increased risk of developing eating disorders, such as anorexia nervosa or bulimia, as individuals resort to extreme measures to achieve the desired body shape or weight. Additionally, body dissatisfaction and negative body image are associated with higher rates of depression, anxiety, and body-related shame and guilt.

5. Self-Worth Tied to Appearance: Unrealistic beauty standards perpetuate the harmful notion that an individual's worth is solely determined by their physical appearance. This emphasis on external validation can undermine one's sense of self-worth and create an unhealthy reliance on external factors for self-esteem and acceptance.

In conclusion, unrealistic beauty standards have a significant impact on body image, contributing to body dissatisfaction and negative self-perception. The internalization of unattainable ideals, distorted body perception, negative body image, and the association of self-worth with appearance all play a role in perpetuating this impact. Promoting a more realistic and inclusive definition of beauty is crucial in fostering body acceptance, improving mental well-being, and nurturing positive body image. Embracing diversity, challenging narrow beauty ideals, and valuing individuality can help individuals develop a healthier and more accepting relationship with their bodies.

Challenging societal norms and promoting body diversity and inclusivity.

Challenging societal norms and promoting body diversity and inclusivity are crucial steps in combating body dissatisfaction and fostering a more positive body image. By challenging narrow beauty ideals and embracing the uniqueness of every individual, we can create a more inclusive and accepting society.

1. Embracing Body Diversity: Society often upholds a limited and unrealistic beauty standard that excludes individuals who do not fit within those narrow parameters. Embracing body diversity means celebrating and appreciating bodies of all shapes, sizes, colors, and abilities. It involves acknowledging that beauty comes in a wide range of forms and that no single body type should be considered superior or more desirable than another.

2. Representation in Media and Advertising: Media and advertising have a significant influence on shaping societal beauty ideals. By advocating for and demanding greater diversity and inclusivity in media representation, we can challenge existing norms and promote body positivity. Encouraging accurate and authentic representation of diverse bodies sends a powerful message that all individuals deserve visibility, respect, and acceptance.

3. Educating on Media Literacy: Promoting media literacy is vital in empowering individuals to critically analyze and challenge unrealistic beauty standards perpetuated by the media. By providing education on media manipulation, photo editing techniques, and the commercial interests behind idealized images, individuals can develop a more

discerning perspective. They can differentiate between fabricated ideals and reality, reducing the negative impact on body image.

4. Redefining Beauty: Challenging societal norms requires redefining beauty on individual terms. It involves shifting the focus from external appearance to qualities like character, kindness, intelligence, and accomplishments. By emphasizing inner qualities, we can break free from the narrow beauty-centric mindset and recognize the multitude of attributes that contribute to true beauty.

5. Promoting Body Positivity: Body positivity is a movement that aims to foster self-acceptance and challenge negative body image. It encourages individuals to embrace their bodies as they are, to celebrate their unique features, and to reject harmful societal judgments. By spreading body positivity, we can create a supportive environment where all bodies are valued, respected, and accepted.

In conclusion, challenging societal norms and promoting body diversity and inclusivity are vital for fostering a more positive body image and combating body dissatisfaction. Embracing body diversity, advocating for accurate representation in media and advertising, promoting media literacy, redefining beauty beyond appearance, and promoting body positivity all contribute to a more inclusive and accepting society. By creating spaces that celebrate and value diverse bodies, we can empower individuals to develop a healthier relationship with their own bodies and promote greater acceptance of others.

Chapter 3

Exploring the psychological factors contributing to body dissatisfaction.

Body dissatisfaction is influenced by various psychological factors that contribute to its development and persistence. Understanding these underlying factors is essential in addressing body dissatisfaction effectively.

1. Social Comparison: Humans have a natural tendency to compare themselves to others, particularly in terms of appearance. Social comparison plays a significant role in body dissatisfaction, as individuals compare their bodies to the perceived "ideal" bodies portrayed in the media or among their peers. This constant comparison can lead to feelings of inadequacy and dissatisfaction with one's own body.

2. Perfectionism: Perfectionistic tendencies contribute to body dissatisfaction as individuals set unrealistically high standards for their appearance. They strive for an idealized body image that is unattainable, leading to chronic dissatisfaction with their own bodies. Perfectionism fuels self-criticism, self-judgment,

and a relentless pursuit of an unrealistic physical ideal.

3. Sociocultural Influences: Societal and cultural factors significantly impact body dissatisfaction. Societal beauty ideals, media portrayals, and cultural norms shape individuals' perceptions of beauty and influence their self-evaluation. Internalizing these standards can lead to negative body image and dissatisfaction when individuals perceive their bodies as not meeting the societal norms.

4. Body-related Shame and Guilt: Feelings of shame and guilt related to one's body can contribute to body dissatisfaction. Negative experiences, body-shaming comments, or internalized beliefs about one's appearance can lead to a deep sense of shame and guilt. These emotions fuel negative self-perception and dissatisfaction with one's body.

5. Body Image Investment: Individuals who invest a significant amount of their self-worth and identity in their physical appearance are more prone to body dissatisfaction. When appearance becomes a primary source of validation and self-esteem, any perceived flaw or deviation from

societal standards can have a disproportionately negative impact on overall well-being.

6. Media Influence: Media plays a substantial role in shaping body dissatisfaction through its portrayal of unrealistic beauty ideals. Constant exposure to idealized and airbrushed images can create distorted perceptions of one's own body and contribute to negative body image. Media literacy is essential in navigating and challenging these influences.

In conclusion, body dissatisfaction is influenced by a range of psychological factors. Social comparison, perfectionism, sociocultural influences, body-related shame and guilt, body image investment, and media influence all contribute to the development and perpetuation of body dissatisfaction. Recognizing and addressing these psychological factors is crucial in promoting body acceptance, nurturing positive self-perception, and improving overall well-being. By fostering self-compassion, challenging unrealistic ideals, and cultivating a healthy relationship with one's body, individuals can work towards a more positive body image and reduced body dissatisfaction.

Discussing the role of self-esteem, self-worth, and identity in body image.

Imagine a young woman named Maya. She has always had a positive outlook on life and exuded confidence in various aspects. However, lately, Maya finds herself struggling with her body image. She compares herself to the idealized bodies she sees in magazines and feels like she falls short. This self-doubt has started to impact her overall self-esteem, self-worth, and sense of identity.

Self-esteem is an individual's overall evaluation of their worth and value. It encompasses how we perceive ourselves, our abilities, and our worthiness. Maya's self-esteem has taken a hit as she begins to question her physical appearance. The negative comparison to unrealistic beauty standards has left her feeling inadequate and doubting her own value.

Self-worth, on the other hand, is a deeper sense of intrinsic value and acceptance of oneself beyond external factors. Maya's self-worth used to be rooted in her unique qualities, achievements, and relationships. However, her recent body image struggles have caused her to question her worthiness as a person. She feels that her body does not meet the societal expectations, leading her to doubt her own worth.

Furthermore, body image can intertwine with an individual's identity. Maya's perception of her body has started to impact how she sees herself as a person. She used to identify with her strengths, passions, and values. However, the focus on her physical appearance has led her to question her identity and whether she can truly be confident and successful if her body doesn't conform to the perceived ideal.

Maya's journey showcases the intricate relationship between self-esteem, self-worth, identity, and body image. When individuals experience dissatisfaction with their bodies, it can erode their self-esteem, leading to self-doubt and a diminished sense of worthiness. It can also affect their identity, as they question how their bodies fit into their self-concept and overall self-image.

In conclusion, self-esteem, self-worth, and identity play vital roles in shaping body image. Negative body image can impact an individual's self-esteem and self-worth, leading to feelings of inadequacy and self-doubt. Moreover, body image struggles can challenge one's sense of identity, as individuals grapple with reconciling their physical appearance with their self-concept. Recognizing and addressing these interconnected aspects is crucial in promoting a healthier and more positive body image. By fostering self-compassion, promoting a holistic sense of self-worth, and embracing diverse identities, individuals can develop a more accepting and positive relationship with their bodies and cultivate a stronger overall sense of self.

Examining the relationship between body image and mental health.

Meet Emily. She has always been a vibrant and outgoing person, but lately, her body image concerns have started to impact her mental health. Emily's journey highlights the complex relationship between body image and mental well-being.

Emily's negative body image has been taking a toll on her mental health. She constantly compares her body to unrealistic beauty standards, feeling inadequate and dissatisfied. This preoccupation with her appearance fuels feelings of anxiety and self-consciousness, affecting her overall emotional well-being.

Body image is intricately linked to mental health. Poor body image can contribute to the development or exacerbation of mental health conditions such as depression, anxiety, and eating disorders. Emily's negative body image has led to symptoms of depression, as she feels a persistent sense of sadness and hopelessness. She also experiences heightened anxiety, constantly worrying about how she is perceived by others and feeling self-conscious in social situations.

Negative body image can also lead to the development of eating disorders. Emily's dissatisfaction with her body has led her to engage in restrictive eating behaviors and obsess over her weight and shape. These behaviors are driven by the belief that achieving an idealized body will bring her happiness and acceptance. This unhealthy relationship with her body has taken a toll on her physical and mental well-being.

Moreover, body image issues can contribute to low self-esteem and self-worth. Emily's negative body image has eroded her self-confidence, causing her to doubt her abilities and value as a person. This diminished self-worth further impacts her mental health, as she struggles with feelings of inadequacy and self-criticism.

Emily's journey exemplifies the significant impact of body image on mental health. Negative body image can contribute to symptoms of depression, anxiety, and eating disorders. It can also erode self-esteem and self-worth, leading to feelings of inadequacy and self-criticism.

Recognizing this relationship is crucial in addressing both body image and mental health concerns. It is important to provide support and interventions that target both aspects concurrently. Encouraging individuals to develop a more positive body image through self-acceptance and challenging societal beauty standards can have a positive impact on their mental well-being.

Emily begins her journey towards healing by seeking professional help. Through therapy, she learns to challenge her negative body image and develop more compassionate and accepting attitudes towards herself. She also receives support for her underlying mental health struggles, working towards recovery from depression and anxiety.

In conclusion, body image and mental health are closely intertwined. Negative body image can contribute to the development or exacerbation of mental health conditions such as depression, anxiety, and eating disorders. It can also erode self-esteem and self-worth, impacting overall emotional well-being. Recognizing and addressing the relationship between body image and mental health is essential in promoting holistic well-being. By fostering self-acceptance, challenging societal beauty standards, and providing support for mental health concerns, individuals can embark on a path towards improved body image and mental well-being.

Chapter 4

Promoting self-acceptance and positive body image.

Promoting self-acceptance and positive body image is crucial in fostering a healthy relationship with one's body and overall well-being. It involves embracing and appreciating oneself as unique and valuable, regardless of societal beauty standards. Here's an explanation of how to promote self-acceptance and positive body image:

1. Cultivating Self-Compassion: Self-compassion involves treating oneself with kindness, understanding, and empathy. It means recognizing that nobody is perfect and that imperfections are a part of being human. By cultivating self-compassion, individuals can develop a more forgiving and accepting attitude towards their bodies, embracing them with kindness and understanding.

2. Challenging Unrealistic Beauty Ideals: Promoting positive body image requires challenging and questioning societal beauty ideals. Encouraging a diverse and inclusive representation of bodies in media, advertising, and popular

culture can help individuals recognize that beauty comes in various shapes, sizes, and forms. By celebrating diverse bodies, we can challenge the notion that there is only one "ideal" body type.

3. Focusing on Health and Well-being: Shifting the focus from appearance-based goals to overall health and well-being can foster a more positive body image. Encouraging individuals to engage in activities they enjoy, eat nourishing foods, and prioritize self-care helps promote a holistic approach to well-being. By prioritizing health, individuals can develop a more positive and balanced perspective on their bodies.

4. Practicing Body Positivity: Body positivity is about celebrating and respecting all bodies, regardless of shape, size, or appearance. It involves adopting a mindset that appreciates the diversity of human bodies and rejects societal judgments based on appearance. Encouraging body-positive language, challenging body-shaming behaviors, and fostering a supportive environment can help individuals develop a more positive body image.

5. Surrounding Oneself with Positive Influences: Surrounding oneself with positive influences can contribute to a healthier body image. Building a

supportive social network that emphasizes self-acceptance, body positivity, and self-care can provide a buffer against negative societal messages. Engaging with body-positive role models, online communities, or support groups can also be beneficial in promoting self-acceptance and positive body image.

6. Practicing Mindfulness and Gratitude: Mindfulness practices can help individuals become more aware of their thoughts and emotions related to their bodies. By practicing self-reflection, individuals can challenge negative thoughts and replace them with positive and empowering affirmations. Additionally, cultivating gratitude for the body's capabilities and focusing on its strengths can foster a more positive body image.

In conclusion, promoting self-acceptance and positive body image involves embracing one's uniqueness, challenging unrealistic beauty ideals, and focusing on overall health and well-being. By cultivating self-compassion, practicing body positivity, surrounding oneself with positive influences, and engaging in mindfulness and gratitude, individuals can develop a healthier and more positive relationship with their bodies. Promoting self-acceptance and positive body image is a continuous journey that requires effort, support, and a commitment to challenging societal norms and embracing diverse definitions of beauty.

Encouraging self-compassion and self-care practices.

Encouraging self-compassion and self-care practices is essential for promoting overall well-being and cultivating a positive relationship with oneself. Here's an explanation of how to encourage self-compassion and self-care:

1. Understanding Self-Compassion: Self-compassion involves treating oneself with kindness, understanding, and non-judgment. It means acknowledging one's own suffering and responding to it with empathy and self-care. Encouraging individuals to understand and embrace self-compassion allows them to develop a more nurturing and supportive relationship with themselves.

2. Practicing Self-Care: Self-care refers to engaging in activities that promote physical, mental, and emotional well-being. Encouraging individuals to prioritize self-care helps them recognize the importance of taking time for themselves and attending to their needs. This can involve engaging

in activities such as exercise, spending time in nature, practicing relaxation techniques, engaging in hobbies, or seeking social support.

3. Setting Boundaries: Encouraging individuals to set boundaries is an important aspect of self-compassion and self-care. This involves recognizing and respecting one's own limits, saying no when necessary, and prioritizing personal well-being. Helping individuals establish healthy boundaries enables them to protect their energy and maintain a balanced and fulfilling life.

4. Nurturing Positive Self-Talk: Encouraging positive self-talk is crucial for fostering self-compassion. By helping individuals become aware of their self-talk patterns and challenging negative self-critical thoughts, they can develop a more positive and supportive inner dialogue. Encouraging affirmations and practicing positive reframing can contribute to building a healthier and more compassionate self-perception.

5. Embracing Mindfulness: Mindfulness practices can enhance self-compassion and self-care. Encouraging individuals to engage in mindfulness activities, such as meditation or deep breathing exercises, helps them become more present in the moment, cultivate self-awareness, and develop a

non-judgmental attitude towards themselves. This fosters a greater sense of self-compassion and the ability to respond to stress and difficulties with kindness and understanding.

6. Seeking Support: Encouraging individuals to seek support when needed is crucial for practicing self-compassion and self-care. This can involve reaching out to trusted friends, family members, or professionals who can provide guidance, empathy, and support. Connecting with others who can offer validation and understanding contributes to overall well-being and fosters a sense of belonging.

In conclusion, encouraging self-compassion and self-care practices is vital for nurturing a positive relationship with oneself. By promoting self-compassion, practicing self-care, setting boundaries, nurturing positive self-talk, embracing mindfulness, and seeking support, individuals can prioritize their well-being and cultivate a compassionate and nurturing relationship with themselves. Encouraging self-compassion and self-care is a powerful way to foster resilience, enhance overall well-being, and promote a healthier and more fulfilling life.

Providing strategies to improve body confidence and self-esteem.

Improving body confidence and self-esteem is a journey that involves cultivating a positive self-perception and developing a healthy relationship with one's body. Here are some strategies to help individuals improve their body confidence and self-esteem:

1. Practice Self-Acceptance: Encourage individuals to embrace their bodies as they are, recognizing that beauty comes in diverse shapes, sizes, and forms. Encouraging self-acceptance involves shifting the focus from external appearance to appreciating the body's strengths, capabilities, and uniqueness. Emphasize the value of self-acceptance as a foundation for building body confidence and self-esteem.

2. Challenge Negative Thoughts: Help individuals identify and challenge negative thoughts related to their bodies. Encourage them to question the validity of these thoughts and replace them with more positive and realistic affirmations. This process involves reframing negative self-talk and focusing on self-compassion and self-love.

3. Cultivate Positive Body Image: Engage individuals in activities that promote positive body image. Encourage them to surround themselves with positive influences, such as body-positive media, affirmations, and supportive social networks. Promote media literacy to help them critically evaluate and challenge unrealistic beauty ideals portrayed in the media.

4. Focus on Health and Well-being: Shifting the focus from appearance to overall health and well-being can improve body confidence and self-esteem. Encourage individuals to engage in activities that promote physical and mental well-being, such as regular exercise, nutritious eating, restful sleep, and stress management. Emphasize the importance of self-care and self-nurturing practices.

5. Celebrate Body Diversity: Encourage individuals to celebrate and appreciate the diversity of bodies. Promote inclusivity and challenge the idea that there is one "ideal" body type. Help them recognize that beauty is not limited to specific physical attributes but is present in the uniqueness of each individual.

6. Set Realistic Goals: Encourage individuals to set realistic goals related to their bodies that are

based on personal health and well-being rather than societal expectations. Help them identify achievable and sustainable changes they can make to support their overall health, allowing them to shift their focus to progress rather than perfection.

7. Seek Support: Encourage individuals to seek support from friends, family, or professionals when working on improving body confidence and self-esteem. Supportive relationships and guidance can provide encouragement, perspective, and validation throughout the process.

8. Practice Self-Care: Promote self-care practices that nurture both the body and mind. Encourage individuals to engage in activities they enjoy, prioritize relaxation, and engage in self-soothing practices. Taking care of oneself holistically fosters a positive self-perception and overall well-being.

In conclusion, improving body confidence and self-esteem requires a combination of self-acceptance, positive body image, a focus on health and well-being, celebrating body diversity, setting realistic goals, seeking support, and practicing self-care. By implementing these strategies, individuals can gradually develop a healthier and more positive relationship with their bodies, leading to increased body confidence and enhanced self-esteem. It is important to remember that this is an ongoing journey, and progress comes with patience, self-compassion, and self-love.

Chapter 5

Addressing the impact of social comparison and peer pressure on body image.

Addressing the impact of social comparison and peer pressure on body image is crucial in promoting a healthier relationship with one's body. Social comparison refers to the tendency of individuals to compare themselves to others, while peer pressure involves the influence exerted by peers to conform to certain standards or behaviors. Here's an explanation of how these factors impact body image:

1. Social Comparison: Humans have a natural inclination to compare themselves to others, particularly in terms of appearance. In today's digital age, social media platforms and the constant exposure to carefully curated images contribute to heightened social comparison. Individuals often compare their bodies to the perceived "ideal" bodies portrayed by influencers, celebrities, or even friends. This constant comparison can lead to feelings of inadequacy and dissatisfaction with one's own body.

2. Unrealistic Beauty Standards: The prevalence of idealized and digitally enhanced images in the media reinforces unrealistic beauty standards. These standards often prioritize thinness, muscularity, and flawless appearance, creating a narrow and unattainable definition of beauty. When individuals compare themselves to these ideals, they may experience body dissatisfaction, as their bodies do not align with the perceived norms.

3. Peer Pressure: Peer pressure can significantly impact body image, as individuals may feel compelled to conform to certain beauty standards to fit in or gain social acceptance. Friends or social circles that emphasize appearance or engage in body-focused conversations or behaviors can contribute to body dissatisfaction. Pressure to conform to specific body ideals can lead to unhealthy dieting, excessive exercise, or engagement in risky behaviors to alter one's appearance.

Addressing the impact of social comparison and peer pressure on body image requires a multi-faceted approach:

1. Promoting Media Literacy: Encouraging individuals to critically evaluate and challenge the

messages portrayed in media is essential. Media literacy education can help individuals recognize the unrealistic nature of many images and understand the digital manipulation that occurs. By fostering a critical mindset, individuals can reduce the negative impact of social comparison and develop a more realistic perspective on beauty.

2. Emphasizing Individuality and Diversity: Highlighting the value of individuality and diversity is important in combating the pressure to conform. Celebrating diverse body shapes, sizes, and appearances promotes inclusivity and challenges the notion of a single idealized body type. By embracing and appreciating individual differences, individuals can develop a more positive and accepting view of their own bodies.

3. Encouraging Positive Peer Influences: Promoting positive peer influences involves fostering supportive and inclusive environments. Encourage open conversations about body image, self-acceptance, and challenging societal beauty standards. By surrounding oneself with friends and communities that prioritize acceptance and celebrate diverse bodies, individuals can reduce the negative impact of peer pressure.

4. Building Self-Esteem and Self-Confidence: Strengthening self-esteem and self-confidence is essential in mitigating the impact of social comparison and peer pressure. Encourage individuals to focus on their unique qualities, strengths, and achievements beyond their appearance. By nurturing self-esteem, individuals become more resilient to external pressures and can develop a more positive body image.

5. Providing Education and Awareness: Promote education and awareness about the harmful effects of social comparison and peer pressure on body image. By providing resources, workshops, or campaigns that address these issues, individuals can gain a better understanding of the impact and develop strategies to navigate societal pressures more effectively.

Addressing the impact of social comparison and peer pressure on body image requires a collective effort. By challenging unrealistic beauty standards, promoting individuality and diversity, fostering positive peer influences, and building self-esteem, we can create a culture that values and respects diverse bodies. Encouraging self-acceptance and self-love becomes key in empowering individuals to navigate social pressures and cultivate a healthier body image.

Discussing strategies for handling societal pressures and negative comments.

Handling societal pressures and negative comments is essential in maintaining a positive body image and preserving one's well-being. Here are some strategies to help individuals navigate and cope with these challenges:

1. Develop Self-Awareness: Cultivating self-awareness allows individuals to recognize when societal pressures or negative comments are affecting their well-being. By becoming aware of their own emotional responses and triggers, individuals can better understand the impact these external factors have on their body image and overall self-perception.

2. Challenge Unrealistic Beauty Standards: Actively challenge societal beauty standards by recognizing their limitations and promoting a more inclusive and diverse definition of beauty. Engage in conversations that challenge unrealistic ideals and emphasize the value of different body shapes, sizes, and appearances. By questioning and challenging these standards, individuals can

reduce their personal investment in meeting narrow societal expectations.

3. Surround Yourself with Positive Influences: Seek out positive and supportive influences in your life. Surround yourself with friends, family, or communities that celebrate and embrace diverse bodies. Engage with media, social media accounts, and influencers that promote body positivity and self-acceptance. Building a network of positive influences can provide encouragement, validation, and support in navigating societal pressures.

4. Practice Self-Compassion: Be kind and compassionate to yourself when faced with negative comments or societal pressures. Acknowledge that negative comments are a reflection of the person making them and not a reflection of your worth or value. Treat yourself with kindness, understanding, and empathy, reminding yourself that you are more than your physical appearance.

5. Set Boundaries: Establish clear boundaries with individuals who consistently make negative comments or contribute to societal pressures. Communicate your boundaries assertively and firmly, emphasizing the importance of respecting and accepting all bodies. Surround yourself with

people who uplift and support you, creating a safe space where negative comments and pressures are minimized.

6. Develop Coping Strategies: Identify healthy coping strategies to manage stress and negative emotions related to societal pressures. This can include engaging in activities that bring joy and boost self-esteem, such as hobbies, exercise, or creative outlets. Practice mindfulness or relaxation techniques to center yourself and reduce anxiety. Seek professional support, such as therapy or counseling, to develop personalized coping strategies and process any negative experiences.

7. Cultivate a Positive Self-Image: Focus on nurturing a positive self-image that extends beyond physical appearance. Embrace your unique qualities, strengths, and accomplishments. Engage in positive self-talk and affirmations to counteract negative comments or self-doubt. Celebrate your body for its functionality, resilience, and the experiences it allows you to have.

8. Educate Others: Share your knowledge and experiences with others to promote understanding and challenge societal pressures collectively. Engage in discussions and advocate

for body positivity, self-acceptance, and inclusivity. By educating others about the harmful effects of negative comments and societal pressures, you can help create a more supportive and accepting environment for all.

Handling societal pressures and negative comments requires resilience, self-awareness, and a strong support system. By challenging beauty standards, surrounding yourself with positive influences, practicing self-compassion, setting boundaries, developing coping strategies, cultivating a positive self-image, and educating others, individuals can navigate these challenges with greater resilience and maintain a positive body image. Remember that your worth extends far beyond societal expectations, and prioritizing your well-being is essential in fostering a healthy relationship with your body.

Promoting assertiveness and setting healthy boundaries

Promoting assertiveness and setting healthy boundaries is crucial for maintaining self-respect, preserving personal well-being, and cultivating positive relationships. Here's an explanation of assertiveness and setting healthy boundaries:

1. Understanding Assertiveness: Assertiveness refers to the ability to express oneself honestly, openly, and confidently, while respecting the rights and boundaries of others. It involves effectively communicating thoughts, feelings, and needs without aggression or passivity. Assertive individuals advocate for themselves while maintaining respect for others.

2. Recognizing Your Rights: Promoting assertiveness starts with recognizing and affirming your rights as an individual. This includes the right to express opinions, make decisions, set boundaries, and prioritize your well-being. Understanding your rights helps build confidence in asserting yourself and setting healthy boundaries in various aspects of life.

3. Identifying Boundaries: Boundaries are personal limits that define what is acceptable and what is not in relationships, interactions, and experiences. They encompass physical, emotional, and mental aspects. Identifying your boundaries involves understanding your comfort levels, needs, and values. It is crucial to recognize that boundaries may vary for different individuals and situations.

4. Communicating Boundaries: Effective communication is key to setting healthy boundaries. Clearly and assertively communicate your boundaries to others, expressing your needs and limits. Use "I" statements to express your feelings and preferences, and be specific about what behaviors or actions are crossing your boundaries. Practice active listening to ensure a mutual understanding in conversations about boundaries.

5. Maintaining Consistency: Consistency is important in setting and maintaining healthy boundaries. Stick to your established boundaries and reinforce them consistently. This helps establish clear expectations for yourself and others, creating a sense of safety and respect within relationships and interactions.

6. Handling Reactions: Be prepared for various reactions when asserting your boundaries. Some individuals may respect and honor your boundaries, while others may push against them or try to manipulate your decision. Stay firm and assertive, validating your own needs and rights. Remember that you have the autonomy to prioritize your well-being.

7. Self-Care and Self-Reflection: Practicing self-care is vital in promoting assertiveness and setting healthy boundaries. Take time for self-reflection to understand your needs, limits, and triggers. Nurture self-compassion and self-esteem, as they form the foundation for advocating for yourself confidently. Engage in activities that promote self-care and recharge your energy.

8. Seek Support: Seek support from trusted friends, family, or professionals who can provide guidance and encouragement in promoting assertiveness and setting healthy boundaries. They can offer perspectives, advice, and validation, especially during challenging situations. Therapy or counseling can also be beneficial for developing assertiveness skills and addressing any underlying issues.

Promoting assertiveness and setting healthy boundaries is a continuous process that requires self-awareness, self-respect, and effective communication. By recognizing your rights, identifying boundaries, communicating them assertively, maintaining consistency, handling reactions, practicing self-care, and seeking support, you can foster healthier relationships, protect your well-being, and cultivate a stronger sense of self. Remember, setting boundaries is an act of self-care and an affirmation of your worth.

Chapter 6

Encouraging holistic well-being beyond physical appearance.

Encouraging holistic well-being beyond physical appearance involves recognizing that a person's overall well-being is not solely determined by their physical attributes, but also by their mental, emotional, and social aspects. Here's an explanation of encouraging holistic well-being:

1. Mental Well-being: Emphasize the importance of mental well-being as an integral part of overall health. Encourage individuals to prioritize their mental health by engaging in activities such as mindfulness, meditation, or therapy. Promote self-reflection, emotional intelligence, and stress management techniques to foster a positive and resilient mindset.

2. Emotional Well-being: Acknowledge and validate emotions as essential components of well-being. Encourage individuals to develop emotional awareness and regulation skills. Promote healthy coping strategies, such as expressing emotions through journaling, creative outlets, or seeking support from friends, family, or

professionals. Foster a safe and non-judgmental environment for emotional expression.

3. Social Connections: Highlight the significance of social connections and relationships for overall well-being. Encourage individuals to foster meaningful connections, engage in supportive friendships, and cultivate a strong support system. Promote empathy, active listening, and effective communication skills to enhance relationships and social interactions.

4. Personal Growth and Fulfillment: Encourage individuals to pursue personal growth and fulfillment in various areas of life, beyond physical appearance. This can involve setting and achieving personal goals, nurturing hobbies and interests, engaging in lifelong learning, or contributing to a larger cause. Supporting individuals in discovering and pursuing their passions helps foster a sense of purpose and fulfillment.

5. Self-Care and Self-Compassion: Promote self-care practices that nurture all aspects of well-being. Encourage individuals to prioritize self-care activities that address their physical, mental, and emotional needs. Advocate for self-compassion, which involves treating oneself with kindness,

understanding, and acceptance during challenging times.

6. Balancing Work-Life Activities: Encourage individuals to strike a balance between work, leisure, and personal life. Support the importance of setting boundaries and allocating time for relaxation, hobbies, and quality time with loved ones. Promote the value of rest, leisure activities, and self-renewal to maintain a well-rounded and fulfilling lifestyle.

7. Mind-Body Connection: Highlight the interplay between the mind and body in overall well-being. Encourage practices such as regular exercise, healthy nutrition, adequate sleep, and stress reduction techniques to support physical health. Emphasize the positive impact of these practices on mental and emotional well-being.

8. Gratitude and Positivity: Foster an attitude of gratitude and positivity. Encourage individuals to cultivate a mindset that focuses on the positive aspects of life, practicing gratitude for what they have and expressing appreciation for themselves and others. This mindset shift contributes to overall well-being and enhances resilience in the face of challenges.

By encouraging holistic well-being beyond physical appearance, individuals can cultivate a more balanced and fulfilling life. Prioritizing mental well-being, emotional health, social connections, personal growth, self-care, work-life balance, and a positive mindset contributes to overall happiness, resilience, and a sense of fulfillment. Emphasizing the value of all these aspects helps individuals develop a more holistic and sustainable approach to well-being.

Exploring self-care practices that promote body and mind nourishment.

Exploring self-care practices that promote body and mind nourishment is a vital aspect of maintaining overall well-being and cultivating a positive relationship with oneself. Here's an explanation of these practices:

1. Physical Activity: Engaging in regular physical activity is an essential form of self-care that nourishes both the body and mind. Exercise releases endorphins, improves mood, reduces stress, and promotes physical health. Whether it's going for a walk, practicing yoga, dancing, or participating in a sport, finding enjoyable and sustainable physical activities can contribute to body and mind nourishment.

2. Mindfulness and Meditation: Incorporating mindfulness and meditation into daily life allows for a deeper connection with oneself. These practices cultivate self-awareness, reduce stress, and promote emotional well-being. Taking moments of stillness to focus on the present moment, observe thoughts without judgment, and practice deep breathing can help calm the mind and bring a sense of tranquility.

3. Restorative Sleep: Prioritizing quality sleep is essential for body and mind nourishment. Create a consistent sleep routine, establish a relaxing environment, and practice good sleep hygiene habits. Quality sleep helps restore energy, enhances cognitive function, supports emotional well-being, and contributes to overall physical health.

4. Nutritious Eating: Nourishing the body with balanced and nutritious meals is an act of self-care. Focus on incorporating whole foods, fruits, vegetables, lean proteins, and healthy fats into your diet. Pay attention to your body's hunger and fullness cues, practice mindful eating, and savor each bite. Strive for a healthy relationship with food that is rooted in nourishment and enjoyment rather than strict rules or deprivation.

5. Relaxation and Stress Management: Engage in activities that promote relaxation and stress management. This can include taking soothing baths, practicing deep breathing exercises, engaging in hobbies, listening to calming music, or spending time in nature. Find what brings you joy and peace, and make time for these activities regularly to reduce stress and nurture your well-being.

6. Creative Expression: Embrace creative outlets as a means of self-expression and self-care. Engaging in activities such as painting, writing, playing music, or crafting allows for the release of emotions, enhances mindfulness, and promotes a sense of fulfillment. Allow yourself the freedom to explore your creativity without judgment or expectations.

7. Social Connections: Cultivating meaningful social connections is an important aspect of self-care. Spend time with loved ones, engage in conversations, and foster relationships that uplift and support you. Surround yourself with individuals who celebrate your uniqueness and contribute positively to your well-being.

8. Seeking Support: Recognize the importance of seeking support when needed. Reach out to

trusted friends, family, or professionals when facing challenges or needing guidance. Therapy or counseling can provide a safe space for exploring emotions, developing coping strategies, and promoting personal growth.

By incorporating these self-care practices into your life, you nourish both your body and mind. Remember that self-care is not a one-size-fits-all approach. Explore and discover what practices resonate with you personally, and create a self-care routine that suits your unique needs and preferences. Prioritizing self-care enables you to nurture your well-being, foster self-compassion, and cultivate a positive and fulfilling relationship with both your body and mind.

Discussing the importance of self-compassion, mindfulness, and stress management.

Self-compassion, mindfulness, and stress management are three interconnected aspects of well-being that play a crucial role in promoting mental and emotional health. Let's explore the importance of each of these elements:

1. Self-Compassion: Self-compassion involves extending kindness, understanding, and

acceptance towards oneself, especially during challenging times. It is about treating oneself with the same care and compassion we would offer to a loved one. Self-compassion is essential because:

- It cultivates a positive self-image: Self-compassion helps individuals develop a healthy and positive relationship with themselves. By recognizing their own worth and acknowledging their struggles with kindness, individuals can foster self-esteem, self-acceptance, and self-love.

- It reduces self-criticism: Self-compassion counteracts the harmful effects of self-criticism and negative self-talk. Rather than berating themselves for perceived shortcomings or mistakes, individuals practice self-compassion by offering understanding and support. This reduces unnecessary stress and promotes a more nurturing inner dialogue.

- It enhances resilience: Self-compassion strengthens resilience by providing individuals with a buffer during difficult times. When facing setbacks or challenges, self-compassion allows individuals to respond with self-care, self-encouragement, and self-validation. It helps individuals bounce back from adversity and cultivate emotional well-being.

2. Mindfulness: Mindfulness is the practice of intentionally focusing one's attention on the present moment, without judgment or attachment. It involves being fully aware of one's thoughts, feelings, bodily sensations, and the surrounding environment. Mindfulness is important because:

 - It cultivates awareness and presence: Mindfulness allows individuals to fully engage with their experiences, promoting a deep sense of presence and connection with the present moment. By being aware of the here and now, individuals can reduce anxiety about the past or future, leading to increased calmness and clarity.

 - It reduces stress and anxiety: Practicing mindfulness helps individuals manage stress and anxiety. By observing thoughts and emotions without judgment, individuals can develop a greater understanding of their inner experiences. This awareness allows for a more measured response to stressors, reducing reactivity and promoting a sense of calm.

 - It enhances overall well-being: Mindfulness contributes to overall well-being by promoting self-awareness, emotional regulation, and improved cognitive function. It helps individuals develop a non-reactive stance towards their thoughts and emotions, fostering a more balanced and compassionate approach to life.

3. Stress Management: Stress management involves adopting strategies and practices to cope with and reduce stress levels. Effective stress management is important because:

 - It protects mental and physical health: Chronic stress can have detrimental effects on both mental and physical health. Engaging in stress management techniques helps individuals mitigate the negative impact of stress, promoting resilience, and reducing the risk of stress-related illnesses.

 - It improves overall well-being: By managing stress effectively, individuals can experience improved overall well-being. Stress management techniques such as relaxation exercises, exercise, time management, and seeking social support can help individuals regain a sense of control, reduce overwhelm, and enhance their quality of life.

 - It promotes balance and self-care: Stress management encourages individuals to prioritize self-care and establish a healthy balance between work, personal life, and relaxation. Engaging in activities that alleviate stress helps individuals replenish their energy, reduce burnout, and maintain their well-being.

By embracing self-compassion, practicing mindfulness, and adopting stress management techniques, individuals can nurture their mental and emotional health. These practices allow for greater self-awareness, reduced self-criticism, improved resilience, increased presence, enhanced stress coping abilities, and an overall sense of well-being. Incorporating these elements into daily life fosters a more compassionate and mindful approach to oneself and others, creating a foundation for long-term psychological and emotional well-being.

Chapter 7

Highlighting the role of relationships and social support in body image.

The role of relationships and social support in body image is significant, as the interactions we have with others can deeply impact how we perceive and feel about our bodies. Here's an explanation of this important role:

1. Validation and Acceptance: Positive relationships can provide validation and acceptance for individuals, reinforcing their sense of self-worth beyond their physical appearance. When friends, family, or partners emphasize qualities beyond looks and prioritize the individual's overall well-being, it promotes a healthier body image. Feeling valued for one's personality, character, and accomplishments fosters a sense of worthiness that extends beyond physical attributes.

2. Peer Influence and Comparison: Peer interactions play a crucial role in shaping body image. Peers can influence body ideals, beauty standards, and appearance-related behaviors. Positive peer influences can support body acceptance, encourage diverse beauty standards,

and promote self-compassion. Conversely, negative peer influences that emphasize unrealistic beauty standards or engage in body-shaming behaviors can contribute to body dissatisfaction and negative self-perceptions.

3. Supportive Conversations: Open and supportive conversations about body image within relationships can be transformative. Sharing experiences, concerns, and vulnerabilities creates a safe space for individuals to express their feelings and challenges related to body image. Supportive partners, friends, or support groups can offer empathy, understanding, and validation, fostering self-acceptance and a sense of belonging.

4. Body Positivity and Inclusivity: Cultivating a body-positive and inclusive social environment is crucial for promoting a healthy body image. Friends, family, and communities that embrace diverse bodies and challenge societal beauty norms create spaces where individuals feel accepted and valued. Encouraging body diversity, celebrating different shapes, sizes, and appearances, and rejecting body shaming or discriminatory attitudes contribute to a positive social atmosphere.

5. Social Media Influence: Social media platforms have become significant influencers of body image. Interactions on these platforms can either promote body positivity or contribute to body dissatisfaction. Following accounts that celebrate diverse bodies, body acceptance, and promote mental well-being can provide a positive social media environment. Actively curating social media feeds to include body-positive content and unfollowing accounts that perpetuate unrealistic beauty standards can have a positive impact on body image.

6. Support during Difficult Times: Relationships and social support become particularly crucial during challenging times related to body image. When individuals face body-related struggles, having supportive friends, family members, or mental health professionals who can provide guidance, empathy, and practical solutions can be invaluable. Seeking professional help through therapy or counseling can offer specialized support in navigating body image issues.

7. Challenging Unrealistic Standards Together: Relationships can become a platform for challenging unrealistic beauty standards and promoting body acceptance. Friends, couples, or communities can engage in discussions,

education, and advocacy that challenge societal norms. By collectively rejecting harmful beauty ideals and promoting inclusivity, individuals can create a positive ripple effect and contribute to a more body-positive society.

Understanding the role of relationships and social support in body image highlights the importance of fostering positive connections and promoting a supportive environment. By cultivating relationships that prioritize acceptance, validation, and inclusive perspectives, individuals can navigate body image challenges with resilience and cultivate a healthier relationship with their bodies. Embracing diverse beauty ideals and promoting body acceptance within our relationships and communities contributes to a more compassionate and empowering society.

Offering advice on fostering positive relationships and supportive communities.

Fostering positive relationships and supportive communities is essential for promoting well-being and cultivating a positive environment. Here's advice on how to nurture these relationships and create a supportive community:

1. Cultivate Empathy and Active Listening: Practice empathy by seeking to understand others' perspectives and experiences without judgment. Engage in active listening, giving your full attention and validating their emotions. Show genuine interest and ask open-ended questions to foster deeper connections and demonstrate that you value their thoughts and feelings.

2. Foster Open Communication: Encourage open and honest communication within your relationships and communities. Create a safe space where individuals feel comfortable expressing their thoughts, concerns, and challenges related to body image or other topics. Promote dialogue that is respectful, non-judgmental, and inclusive.

3. Embrace Diversity and Inclusivity: Value and celebrate diversity in all its forms, including body diversity. Recognize that everyone's journey and experiences are unique. Embrace individuals from different backgrounds, body shapes, sizes, and appearances. Challenge stereotypes and biases, fostering a sense of inclusivity and respect for all.

4. Reject Body Shaming and Discrimination: Take a stand against body shaming, discriminatory language, and behavior. Promote body positivity

and challenge harmful beauty ideals. Encourage others to refrain from making negative comments about their own or others' bodies. Foster an environment where individuals feel safe and accepted, regardless of their physical appearance.

5. Provide Support and Validation: Be a source of support for others by offering encouragement, validation, and empathy. Acknowledge their feelings and experiences related to body image challenges. Offer practical help or resources when appropriate. Show that you are there for them, fostering a sense of trust and mutual support.

6. Engage in Education and Awareness: Promote education and awareness about body image issues and the impact of societal pressures. Share resources, articles, or books that challenge beauty standards and promote body acceptance. Engage in conversations and workshops that foster understanding and empathy. Encourage continuous learning and growth within your community.

7. Practice Collaboration and Cooperation: Foster a sense of collaboration and cooperation within your relationships and communities. Encourage individuals to work together towards common goals, such as promoting body positivity or

challenging societal norms. Recognize that collective efforts can bring about meaningful change and support one another in these endeavors.

8. Lead by Example: Be a positive role model by embodying self-acceptance, self-compassion, and body positivity. Practice self-care and demonstrate healthy behaviors that prioritize overall well-being. Show others that it is possible to cultivate a positive relationship with their bodies and promote a supportive community.

9. Seek Professional Help if Needed: If you or others are facing significant challenges related to body image, mental health, or self-esteem, encourage seeking professional help. Mental health professionals can provide specialized support and guidance in navigating these issues. Encourage individuals to prioritize their well-being and seek the help they need without judgment or stigma.

By following these guidelines, you can contribute to the creation of positive relationships and supportive communities. Remember, fostering such an environment takes time and effort. Be patient, practice kindness, and lead with empathy. Together, we can build a world where individuals feel accepted, supported, and empowered in their journey towards body acceptance and overall well-being.

Discussing how to address body image concerns within families, friendships, and romantic partnerships.

Addressing body image concerns within families, friendships, and romantic partnerships can be challenging but crucial for fostering understanding, support, and a healthy body image. Here's an explanation of how to approach these conversations:

1. Create a Safe and Judgment-Free Space: Start by creating a safe and non-judgmental environment where individuals feel comfortable discussing body image concerns. Emphasize that the purpose of the conversation is to support and understand each other, rather than to critique or fix. Set the tone by listening attentively, responding empathetically, and respecting each person's experiences and feelings.

2. Practice Active Listening and Empathy: Approach these discussions with a genuine desire to understand the other person's perspective. Practice active listening by giving your full

attention, maintaining eye contact, and asking clarifying questions. Show empathy by validating their feelings, acknowledging their experiences, and expressing understanding. Avoid making dismissive or judgmental comments.

3. Promote Body Positivity and Self-Acceptance: Encourage a mindset that emphasizes self-acceptance and body positivity within your relationships. Share messages and resources that challenge societal beauty standards and promote a diverse and inclusive definition of beauty. Engage in activities or discussions that highlight and celebrate each person's unique qualities, talents, and accomplishments beyond physical appearance.

4. Focus on Health and Functionality: Shift the focus from solely appearance-based discussions to a broader perspective on health and functionality. Encourage conversations about overall well-being, such as engaging in activities that promote physical fitness, mental health, and emotional well-being. Emphasize the importance of self-care, healthy habits, and balanced lifestyles rather than solely pursuing a specific body shape or size.

5. Avoid Body Shaming and Negative Comments: Be mindful of the language used within your

relationships and avoid body shaming or making negative comments about your own or others' bodies. Instead, foster an environment that values and supports body diversity, emphasizing the importance of self-love, self-compassion, and self-acceptance.

6. Educate and Share Information: Provide educational resources about body image, media literacy, and the societal factors that influence our perceptions of beauty. Share articles, books, documentaries, or social media accounts that challenge unrealistic beauty ideals and promote body acceptance. Encourage open discussions and learning together as a way to promote understanding and support.

7. Seek Professional Help if Needed: If body image concerns are deeply rooted or causing significant distress, consider seeking professional help. A qualified therapist or counselor can provide guidance, support, and strategies for navigating these challenges within family, friendship, or romantic contexts. Encourage and support each other in seeking professional assistance when necessary.

8. Lead by Example: Be mindful of your own attitudes and behaviors towards your body and

demonstrate self-acceptance and body positivity. Engage in healthy habits, practice self-care, and foster a positive relationship with your own body. By leading by example, you can inspire and encourage others to develop a healthier body image.

Addressing body image concerns within families, friendships, and romantic partnerships requires open communication, empathy, and a commitment to creating a supportive environment. These conversations may be difficult, but by fostering understanding, promoting body positivity, and prioritizing each person's well-being, you can build stronger, more supportive relationships that contribute to a healthier body image for everyone involved.

Chapter 8

Recognizing when body dissatisfaction becomes severe and impacts mental health.

Recognizing when body dissatisfaction becomes severe and impacts mental health is crucial for early intervention and support. Body dissatisfaction can manifest in varying degrees, but when it reaches a severe level, it can have significant consequences on a person's mental and emotional well-being. Here's an explanation of this recognition process:

1. Persistent Negative Thoughts and Feelings: Severe body dissatisfaction often involves persistent negative thoughts and feelings about one's appearance. These thoughts may be intrusive, overwhelming, and difficult to control. The individual may engage in excessive self-criticism, comparing themselves unfavorably to others, and experiencing a constant sense of dissatisfaction or disgust with their body.

2. Preoccupation with Appearance: When body dissatisfaction becomes severe, it can lead to an excessive preoccupation with appearance. The individual may spend an excessive amount of time

and energy on appearance-related activities, such as checking their reflection repeatedly, engaging in extensive grooming rituals, or constantly seeking validation from others about their appearance.

3. Emotional Distress and Impaired Functioning: Severe body dissatisfaction often accompanies significant emotional distress. The individual may experience heightened levels of anxiety, depression, or low self-esteem. These negative emotions can impact various aspects of their life, such as relationships, social interactions, work or school performance, and overall quality of life.

4. Disordered Eating Behaviors: In some cases, severe body dissatisfaction can contribute to disordered eating behaviors, such as restrictive eating, binge eating, or engaging in unhealthy weight control measures. These behaviors may be driven by a desperate desire to attain a specific body shape or size, leading to an unhealthy relationship with food and potential physical health complications.

5. Social Withdrawal and Isolation: Severe body dissatisfaction can lead to social withdrawal and isolation. The individual may avoid social situations, intimate relationships, or activities that involve exposing their body. They may feel self-

conscious or believe that others are judging them based on their appearance, leading to a withdrawal from social connections and a reduced quality of life.

6. Impact on Mental Health: Severe body dissatisfaction can significantly impact mental health, leading to conditions such as body dysmorphic disorder, eating disorders, depression, anxiety disorders, or other related mental health conditions. It is essential to recognize the potential signs and symptoms of these disorders and seek professional help when needed.

If you or someone you know is experiencing severe body dissatisfaction and it is impacting mental health, it is crucial to seek support from mental health professionals. They can provide a comprehensive assessment, diagnosis, and appropriate treatment options tailored to the individual's specific needs. Treatment may involve therapy, counseling, support groups, or a combination of interventions to address the underlying issues and promote healing and recovery.

By recognizing when body dissatisfaction reaches a severe level and impacts mental health, individuals can take the necessary steps towards seeking help, receiving support, and embarking on a journey towards healing and improved well-being. Remember, early intervention is key, and there is support available to guide individuals through this challenging time.

Providing information on seeking professional assistance, such as therapists or counselors.

Seeking professional assistance, such as therapists or counselors, is an important step when facing challenges related to body image, self-esteem, and mental health. Here's an explanation of the process and benefits of seeking professional help:

1. Recognizing the Need for Support: The first step in seeking professional assistance is recognizing that you or someone you know could benefit from additional support. This recognition may come from experiencing persistent body dissatisfaction, significant distress, impaired functioning, or the inability to cope effectively with related emotions and challenges.

2. Researching and Choosing a Professional: Once you've recognized the need for support, it's important to research and choose a qualified professional who specializes in the specific area of concern. Look for therapists or counselors who have experience in body image issues, self-esteem, eating disorders, or related mental health conditions. Seek recommendations from trusted sources, consult online directories, or contact mental health organizations for guidance.

3. Initial Consultation and Assessment: The first session with a therapist or counselor typically involves an initial consultation and assessment. This is an opportunity to discuss your concerns, goals, and any relevant background information. The professional will ask questions to gain a deeper understanding of your experiences and provide an initial evaluation of your needs.

4. Tailored Treatment Approach: Based on the assessment, the therapist or counselor will develop a personalized treatment plan to address your specific concerns. This plan may involve various therapeutic techniques, such as cognitive-behavioral therapy (CBT), dialectical behavior therapy (DBT), mindfulness-based approaches, or other evidence-based interventions. The

treatment approach will be tailored to your unique circumstances and needs.

5. Individual or Group Therapy: Therapy can be conducted in individual or group settings, depending on your preference and the recommendations of the professional. Individual therapy provides one-on-one sessions where you can explore your concerns, emotions, and thought patterns in a private and confidential environment. Group therapy involves joining a supportive group of individuals facing similar challenges, providing opportunities for shared experiences, insights, and peer support.

6. Confidentiality and Safe Space: Professional therapists and counselors adhere to strict ethical guidelines, ensuring confidentiality and creating a safe space for open and honest discussions. They provide a non-judgmental and supportive environment where you can freely express your thoughts, emotions, and concerns without fear of judgment or disclosure.

7. Collaborative and Supportive Relationship: Therapy involves building a collaborative and supportive relationship with your therapist or counselor. They serve as a guide and ally in your journey towards healing and personal growth.

Through active listening, empathy, and expertise, they help you explore underlying issues, develop coping strategies, challenge negative beliefs, and promote positive change.

8. Continuity and Progress: Therapy is typically conducted over a series of sessions, and the frequency and duration will depend on your specific needs. It's important to attend sessions consistently and actively engage in the therapeutic process. Over time, therapy can lead to increased self-awareness, improved coping skills, enhanced self-esteem, and a more positive body image.

9. Ongoing Support and Aftercare: Seeking professional assistance is not just a short-term solution but a step towards long-term well-being. After completing therapy, it is important to maintain the progress made and continue practicing the strategies learned. Your therapist or counselor may provide you with tools, resources, or recommendations for ongoing self-care and support.

Remember, seeking professional assistance is a courageous and empowering step towards taking care of your mental health. It allows you to work with a trained professional who can offer guidance, support, and evidence-based interventions tailored to your specific needs. By seeking help, you're investing in your well-being and embarking on a journey of self-discovery, healing, and personal growth.

Exploring evidence-based interventions and therapies for body image concerns.

Exploring evidence-based interventions and therapies for body image concerns can provide individuals with effective strategies and support for improving their body image and overall well-being. Here's an explanation of some commonly used approaches:

1. Cognitive-Behavioral Therapy (CBT): CBT is a widely recognized and effective therapy for body image concerns. It focuses on identifying and challenging negative thoughts and beliefs related to body image. CBT helps individuals develop healthier and more realistic perspectives on their bodies, challenge distorted thinking patterns, and develop coping strategies to manage negative emotions and behaviors.

2. Acceptance and Commitment Therapy (ACT): ACT combines mindfulness and acceptance-based strategies to help individuals develop a more compassionate and accepting attitude towards

their bodies. It encourages individuals to focus on their values and commit to actions that align with their values rather than being driven solely by appearance-related concerns. ACT helps individuals cultivate psychological flexibility and develop a more positive relationship with their bodies.

3. Body Image Group Therapy: Group therapy specifically designed for body image concerns can be highly beneficial. Group therapy provides a supportive and non-judgmental environment where individuals can share their experiences, gain insights from others, and receive validation and support. Group therapy fosters a sense of belonging and reduces feelings of isolation by realizing that others face similar challenges.

4. Dialectical Behavior Therapy (DBT): DBT combines mindfulness, emotion regulation, distress tolerance, and interpersonal effectiveness skills. While initially developed for borderline personality disorder, DBT has also shown efficacy in addressing body image concerns. It helps individuals develop skills to manage distressing emotions, regulate their emotional responses, and improve interpersonal relationships.

5. Mindfulness-Based Interventions: Mindfulness-based interventions, such as Mindfulness-Based Stress Reduction (MBSR) or Mindfulness-Based Cognitive Therapy (MBCT), can be beneficial for body image concerns. These interventions involve cultivating present-moment awareness, non-judgmental observation of thoughts and emotions, and developing self-compassion. Mindfulness practices can help individuals become more accepting of their bodies and reduce critical self-evaluation.

6. Expressive Therapies: Expressive therapies, such as art therapy or dance/movement therapy, can provide alternative ways of expressing and exploring body image concerns. These creative approaches allow individuals to engage with their bodies in a non-verbal and expressive manner, fostering self-expression, self-awareness, and self-acceptance.

7. Self-Compassion-Based Interventions: Interventions focused on promoting self-compassion can be beneficial for improving body image. These interventions aim to cultivate kindness, understanding, and acceptance towards oneself. They involve learning to treat oneself with the same compassion and care that one would

offer to a friend, promoting self-acceptance and nurturing a positive self-image.

It's important to note that the selection of an evidence-based intervention or therapy depends on an individual's specific needs, preferences, and the expertise of the mental health professional. A qualified therapist or counselor can provide a comprehensive assessment and recommend the most suitable approach tailored to the individual.

By engaging in evidence-based interventions and therapies, individuals can gain valuable tools and strategies to navigate body image concerns, challenge negative thoughts and beliefs, and develop a more positive and compassionate relationship with their bodies. These interventions provide support, guidance, and a framework for personal growth and well-being.

Chapter 9

Discussing the body positivity movement and its impact on self-acceptance.

The body positivity movement has had a significant impact on promoting self-acceptance and challenging societal beauty norms. Here's an explanation of the movement and its influence:

1. Redefining Beauty Standards: The body positivity movement aims to challenge narrow and unrealistic beauty standards imposed by society. It emphasizes that all bodies, regardless of size, shape, color, or ability, are worthy of acceptance and celebration. By broadening the definition of beauty, the movement encourages individuals to appreciate the diversity of human bodies and reject the idea that there is a single "ideal" body type.

2. Fostering Self-Acceptance and Self-Love: Body positivity promotes self-acceptance and self-love, encouraging individuals to embrace and appreciate their own bodies. It aims to shift the focus from appearance-based validation to recognizing and valuing one's inherent worth, beyond physical attributes. This shift promotes a

more compassionate and nurturing relationship with oneself, allowing individuals to develop a positive body image and higher levels of self-esteem.

3. Empowering Marginalized Groups: The body positivity movement particularly addresses the marginalization and discrimination experienced by individuals whose bodies have been historically stigmatized, such as those in larger bodies, people of color, disabled individuals, and the LGBTQ+ community. By giving a voice to these marginalized groups, the movement aims to challenge the oppressive beauty standards that perpetuate exclusion and discrimination.

4. Advocating for Inclusivity and Representation: Body positivity advocates for inclusivity and representation in media, advertising, and other platforms. It calls for a more diverse and realistic portrayal of bodies, encouraging the inclusion of individuals from different backgrounds, sizes, ages, and abilities. Increased representation allows individuals to see themselves reflected positively in society, fostering a sense of belonging and acceptance.

5. Encouraging Self-Expression and Individuality: The body positivity movement recognizes and

celebrates the uniqueness of each individual. It encourages self-expression and the freedom to explore personal style, fashion choices, and other forms of body adornment without judgment or societal pressure. By embracing individuality, the movement promotes self-expression as an essential aspect of self-acceptance and body positivity.

6. Challenging Harmful Beauty Standards: The body positivity movement challenges harmful beauty practices, such as extreme dieting, cosmetic surgeries, or harmful weight loss behaviors. It advocates for a shift towards health-focused behaviors, body autonomy, and self-care practices that prioritize overall well-being rather than conforming to societal beauty standards.

7. Promoting Intersectionality: The body positivity movement recognizes that body image concerns intersect with other forms of oppression and discrimination. It promotes intersectionality by acknowledging that body image struggles can vary based on factors such as race, gender identity, socioeconomic status, and more. Intersectional body positivity aims to create a more inclusive and equitable movement that addresses the unique challenges faced by different communities.

Overall, the body positivity movement has had a transformative impact on self-acceptance by challenging societal beauty norms, promoting inclusivity, and empowering individuals to embrace their bodies. By encouraging self-love, fostering a sense of belonging, and advocating for representation, the movement has created a platform for individuals to challenge negative body image and cultivate a more positive, accepting, and compassionate relationship with their own bodies.

Encouraging readers to participate in body positivity activism.

Encouraging readers to participate in body positivity activism is an empowering call to action that can contribute to positive change in society. Here's an explanation of how individuals can engage in body positivity activism:

1. Educate Yourself: Start by educating yourself about body positivity, its core principles, and its impact on individuals and communities. Learn about the experiences of marginalized groups and the intersections of body image concerns with other forms of oppression. Read books, articles,

and listen to podcasts or watch documentaries that explore body positivity and related topics.

2. Challenge Internalized Bias: Reflect on your own beliefs, attitudes, and biases about body image. Recognize and challenge any internalized negative messages you may have absorbed from societal beauty norms. Work on embracing a more inclusive and accepting mindset, free from judgments about yourself and others based on appearance.

3. Promote Inclusivity and Representation: Actively seek out and support diverse representations of bodies in media, advertising, and other platforms. Amplify voices from marginalized communities and encourage inclusive representation in these spaces. Support brands, influencers, and content creators who prioritize diversity and promote body positivity.

4. Engage in Positive Self-Talk: Practice positive self-talk and encourage others to do the same. Promote affirming messages about body acceptance and self-love. Share positive and empowering content on social media and challenge negative or body-shaming conversations online.

5. Support Body-Positive Initiatives: Engage with organizations, campaigns, or initiatives that promote body positivity and self-acceptance. Donate to or volunteer for organizations working to challenge harmful beauty standards, promote inclusivity, and provide support for individuals struggling with body image issues.

6. Advocate for Change: Speak up against body shaming, discrimination, and harmful beauty practices. Use your voice to challenge oppressive beauty norms and advocate for policies and practices that promote inclusivity, diversity, and body acceptance. Engage in conversations with friends, family, and peers to raise awareness and promote positive change.

7. Foster Supportive Communities: Create or contribute to supportive communities that prioritize body positivity and acceptance. Surround yourself with individuals who uplift and support each other in their body image journeys. Organize or participate in body-positive events, workshops, or support groups that foster a sense of belonging and self-empowerment.

8. Practice Self-Care and Self-Compassion: Engage in self-care practices that prioritize your well-being and promote self-acceptance. Nourish your body

with healthy choices, engage in activities that bring joy and fulfillment, and cultivate self-compassion. By taking care of yourself, you become a role model for others and contribute to a culture of self-care and body positivity.

Remember, body positivity activism is a collective effort, and every individual can make a difference. By participating in body positivity activism, you contribute to the larger movement of challenging harmful beauty standards, promoting inclusivity, and fostering a more accepting and compassionate society. Your actions and advocacy have the power to inspire and empower others, creating a ripple effect of positive change.

Exploring ways to challenge societal beauty norms and promote inclusivity.

Exploring ways to challenge societal beauty norms and promote inclusivity is essential for fostering a more accepting and diverse society. Here's an explanation of how individuals can engage in this important work:

1. Reflect on Personal Biases: Start by reflecting on your own biases and assumptions about beauty. Consider how societal beauty norms have influenced your perceptions and attitudes.

Challenge and question these biases to develop a more inclusive mindset that appreciates diverse appearances and rejects narrow beauty ideals.

2. Embrace Self-Acceptance: Cultivate self-acceptance by recognizing and appreciating your own unique qualities and characteristics beyond physical appearance. Focus on your strengths, talents, and achievements, and practice self-compassion. By embracing self-acceptance, you can inspire others to do the same and challenge the notion that worth is solely tied to external appearance.

3. Promote Media Literacy: Develop media literacy skills to critically analyze and challenge beauty ideals presented in mainstream media. Be mindful of the images and messages you consume, and question their impact on body image. Share resources and engage in conversations about media representation and its influence on societal beauty norms.

4. Support Inclusive Brands and Businesses: Choose to support brands and businesses that promote inclusivity, diversity, and body positivity. Seek out companies that feature a range of body types, ethnicities, genders, and abilities in their marketing and advertising. By using your

consumer power, you send a message to the industry that inclusivity matters.

5. Amplify Marginalized Voices: Actively seek out and amplify the voices of marginalized individuals and communities that challenge societal beauty norms. Share their stories, artwork, and perspectives through social media, blogs, or other platforms. By elevating these voices, you contribute to a more inclusive narrative and help diversify the beauty standards represented in society.

6. Advocate for Policy Changes: Support policy changes that promote inclusivity, such as regulations on unrealistic photo manipulation in advertising or promoting diversity in media representation. Get involved in advocacy campaigns or sign petitions that aim to challenge harmful beauty practices and promote a more inclusive and diverse society.

7. Educate Others: Share your knowledge and insights about societal beauty norms and their impact on individuals. Engage in conversations with friends, family, and colleagues to raise awareness and promote understanding. Offer resources, articles, or books that explore body

image, self-esteem, and inclusivity to spark discussions and encourage critical thinking.

8. Foster Inclusive Conversations: Create a safe and inclusive space for conversations about beauty and body image. Encourage open dialogue that celebrates diversity, challenges stereotypes, and promotes self-acceptance. Actively listen to others' experiences and perspectives, fostering empathy and understanding.

9. Lead by Example: Model inclusive behaviors and attitudes in your daily life. Embrace diversity in your social circles, challenge body-shaming comments, and celebrate individuality. By leading by example, you inspire others to question beauty norms and promote inclusivity in their own lives.

Challenging societal beauty norms and promoting inclusivity requires ongoing effort and a commitment to change. By engaging in these practices, individuals can contribute to a more accepting, diverse, and compassionate society where all bodies are valued and celebrated. Remember, every small action counts and can have a ripple effect of positive change.

Chapter 10

Providing strategies for maintaining a positive body image in the face of challenges.

Maintaining a positive body image in the face of challenges can be a journey that requires self-care, self-compassion, and conscious effort. Here are some strategies that can help:

1. Practice Self-Reflection: Take time to reflect on your thoughts and beliefs about your body. Identify any negative or critical self-talk and challenge those thoughts with more positive and realistic perspectives. Remind yourself of your worth beyond your physical appearance, focusing on your qualities, talents, and achievements.

2. Surround Yourself with Positive Influences: Surround yourself with positive influences that promote body positivity and self-acceptance. Seek out social media accounts, books, podcasts, or communities that celebrate diverse bodies and challenge societal beauty norms. Create an environment that uplifts and inspires you.

3. Cultivate Self-Care Habits: Engage in self-care practices that prioritize your overall well-being. This can include activities like exercise, getting enough sleep, nourishing your body with nutritious food, and engaging in activities that bring you joy and fulfillment. Taking care of yourself holistically can improve your self-image and overall happiness.

4. Practice Mindfulness: Incorporate mindfulness practices into your daily routine. This can include activities like meditation, deep breathing exercises, or simply being present in the moment. Mindfulness helps you develop a non-judgmental and accepting attitude towards your body, cultivating a sense of gratitude for all that it allows you to experience.

5. Surround Yourself with Supportive People: Surround yourself with friends, family, or a support group who value you for who you are beyond your appearance. Seek out relationships that prioritize kindness, respect, and acceptance. Having a strong support network can provide a safe space to express your concerns and receive support and validation.

6. Set Realistic and Personal Goals: Instead of focusing solely on changing your body, set realistic

and personal goals that are unrelated to appearance. Shift your focus to achievements, personal growth, and cultivating meaningful connections. This helps to broaden your sense of self-worth beyond physical attributes.

7. Challenge Comparison and Social Media Influence: Be mindful of the impact of comparison and social media on your body image. Limit exposure to images or content that triggers negative feelings or comparison. Remind yourself that social media often presents curated and idealized versions of reality. Focus on your own journey and celebrate your unique qualities.

8. Practice Self-Compassion: Treat yourself with kindness, compassion, and understanding. Acknowledge that everyone has imperfections and that it is normal to have body insecurities. When facing challenges, practice self-compassion by speaking to yourself as you would to a close friend, offering support and encouragement.

9. Seek Professional Help if Needed: If body image concerns are significantly impacting your mental well-being, consider seeking professional help. A therapist or counselor can provide specialized support and guide you through techniques and

interventions to improve body image and self-esteem.

Remember, developing a positive body image is a process that takes time and patience. Be gentle with yourself and embrace the uniqueness of your own body. By implementing these strategies and seeking support when needed, you can foster a positive and healthy relationship with your body, allowing you to thrive and enjoy life to the fullest.

Addressing setbacks and relapses in body acceptance.

Addressing setbacks and relapses in body acceptance is an important aspect of the journey towards developing a positive body image. It is common to experience ups and downs, and setbacks should be viewed as opportunities for growth and learning. Here's an explanation of how to address setbacks and relapses in body acceptance:

1. Normalize Setbacks: Recognize that setbacks and relapses are a normal part of any transformative process, including the journey towards body acceptance. It is common to have moments of self-doubt, comparison, or negative

self-talk. Avoid being too hard on yourself and understand that setbacks do not define your progress or worth.

2. Practice Self-Compassion: Be kind and compassionate towards yourself during setbacks. Treat yourself with the same kindness and understanding you would offer to a close friend who is going through a difficult time. Remind yourself that setbacks are opportunities for growth and that it is okay to stumble along the way.

3. Reflect on Triggers and Patterns: Take some time to reflect on the triggers or patterns that may have contributed to the setback. Identify any negative influences, situations, or thoughts that may have influenced your body acceptance journey. This reflection can help you develop strategies to better navigate similar situations in the future.

4. Challenge Negative Thoughts: When faced with negative thoughts or self-criticism, challenge them with more realistic and compassionate perspectives. Reframe negative thoughts into positive and affirming statements. Remind yourself of your progress, your worth beyond appearance, and the reasons why you embarked

on the journey towards body acceptance in the first place.

5. Seek Support: Reach out to your support system during setbacks. Share your feelings, concerns, and struggles with trusted friends, family, or a therapist. Talking about your experience can provide you with validation, different perspectives, and support, reminding you that you are not alone in your journey.

6. Engage in Self-Care: Prioritize self-care during setbacks. Engage in activities that promote relaxation, self-soothing, and self-nurturing. This may include practicing mindfulness, taking a break from triggering environments or media, engaging in hobbies or activities that bring you joy, or seeking professional help if needed.

7. Adjust Goals and Expectations: Assess whether your goals and expectations regarding body acceptance are realistic and sustainable. It may be necessary to adjust your goals or revisit your expectations to ensure they align with your values and overall well-being. Focus on progress rather than perfection and celebrate small victories along the way.

8. Learn from Setbacks: View setbacks as learning opportunities. Reflect on what you can learn from the setback and how you can apply these insights to your ongoing journey of body acceptance. Consider what strategies or resources could be helpful in overcoming similar challenges in the future.

Remember, setbacks and relapses are natural, and progress in body acceptance is not linear. Be patient with yourself and celebrate the courage it takes to continue working towards a positive body image. By acknowledging setbacks, practicing self-compassion, seeking support, and learning from the experience, you can navigate through setbacks and continue on your path towards body acceptance and self-love.

Offering guidance on embracing body acceptance as a lifelong journey.

Embracing body acceptance as a lifelong journey is an ongoing process that involves continuous self-reflection, self-care, and self-compassion. Here's an explanation of how to approach and navigate this journey:

1. Shift the Focus: Instead of aiming for a destination or a specific endpoint in your body

acceptance journey, shift your focus to the present moment. Embrace the process and the growth that occurs along the way. Understand that body acceptance is not a one-time achievement but an ongoing practice.

2. Cultivate Self-Reflection: Engage in regular self-reflection to deepen your understanding of yourself and your relationship with your body. Explore your thoughts, feelings, and beliefs about body image. Identify any internalized societal pressures or negative self-talk that may be hindering your progress. Continuously question and challenge those beliefs to foster self-acceptance.

3. Practice Self-Care: Prioritize self-care practices that nourish both your body and mind. Engage in activities that promote overall well-being, such as exercise, healthy eating, adequate rest, and engaging in activities that bring you joy and fulfillment. Taking care of yourself holistically supports your body acceptance journey.

4. Embrace Mindfulness: Incorporate mindfulness practices into your daily life. Cultivate present-moment awareness, non-judgment, and self-compassion. Be attuned to your body's sensations, thoughts, and emotions without attaching

judgment or criticism. Mindfulness helps you develop a deeper connection with your body and cultivates acceptance.

5. Surround Yourself with Positive Influences: Surround yourself with individuals, communities, and resources that promote body positivity and self-acceptance. Seek out supportive social circles, read books and articles that inspire body acceptance, and engage with content that celebrates diverse bodies. Surrounding yourself with positive influences reinforces and sustains your commitment to body acceptance.

6. Practice Gratitude: Cultivate a sense of gratitude for your body and all that it allows you to experience. Shift your focus from perceived flaws to appreciating your body's capabilities, strengths, and resilience. Regularly express gratitude for your body through affirmations or journaling to foster a more positive and appreciative mindset.

7. Embrace Progress, Not Perfection: Understand that body acceptance is not about achieving a perfect body or eliminating all insecurities. Instead, focus on progress and personal growth. Celebrate small victories, acknowledge the steps

you've taken, and appreciate the positive changes you've made along your journey.

8. Seek Support: Surround yourself with a supportive network of friends, family, or a community that shares your commitment to body acceptance. Seek professional help if needed, such as therapy or counseling, to gain additional guidance and support. Having a supportive network can provide encouragement, validation, and resources to navigate challenges and setbacks.

9. Practice Self-Compassion: Be gentle and compassionate with yourself throughout your journey. Treat yourself with kindness, understanding, and patience. When faced with setbacks or difficulties, offer yourself words of encouragement and remind yourself that this is a lifelong process. Embrace self-compassion as an essential component of your body acceptance journey.

Remember, embracing body acceptance as a lifelong journey requires dedication, patience, and self-compassion. Be open to learning and growing, and allow yourself to evolve along the way. Embrace the beauty and uniqueness of your own body, and celebrate the progress you make as you continue to nurture a positive and accepting relationship with it.

Final Words

In this book, we have explored the deep-rooted issues of body dissatisfaction, self-esteem struggles, and societal pressures that many individuals face. But amidst the challenges, there is hope, support, and a wealth of positive help available to you. This book serves as a guiding light, offering insights, strategies, and evidence-based interventions to empower you on your journey towards self-acceptance and body positivity.

You are not alone in your struggles. Countless others have faced similar challenges and have found strength, healing, and growth. By delving into the narratives and research presented in this book, you will gain a deeper understanding of the psychological, social, and cultural factors that contribute to body dissatisfaction. You will explore strategies to challenge societal norms, foster self-compassion, and develop a positive body image.

Through chapters that address various aspects of body image, self-esteem, relationships, and self-care, you will find practical tools, empowering exercises, and real-life stories that resonate with your experiences. The book emphasizes the importance of self-reflection, self-care, and surrounding yourself with a supportive community. It encourages you to embrace your uniqueness, challenge societal beauty standards, and celebrate body diversity.

Remember, your journey towards self-acceptance and body positivity is not linear. There may be setbacks and relapses along the way, but these are opportunities for growth and learning. Take comfort in the fact that setbacks do not define your progress or worth. With self-compassion and resilience, you can navigate through these challenges and continue to move forward.

You have the power to rewrite your narrative and cultivate a positive relationship with your body. Each step you take, no matter how small, contributes to your overall well-being and creates a ripple effect of positive change. As you embark on this transformative journey, embrace self-care, seek support, and celebrate your victories, no matter how seemingly insignificant they may appear.

Remember, you are deserving of love, respect, and acceptance just as you are. You are more than your appearance. Your worth extends far beyond societal beauty standards. You have the strength within you to overcome self-doubt, societal pressures, and negative self-talk. Embrace the power of self-acceptance, cultivate a positive body image, and live a life that is authentically yours.

This book is a testament to the incredible strength and resilience of the human spirit. May it guide you, inspire you, and provide you with the tools and insights needed to embark on a journey of self-discovery, self-love, and body acceptance. You have the power to transform your relationship with your body and embrace a life filled with joy, confidence, and inner peace. Believe in yourself, for you are capable of incredible things.

Things of interest

What does the bible tell us?

The Bible does not explicitly address body image as a specific topic. However, it does provide principles and teachings that can guide our understanding and approach to body image. Here are some key points that can be derived from biblical teachings:

1. God's Creation and Value: The Bible teaches that every individual is fearfully and wonderfully made by God (Psalm 139:14). Our bodies are seen as valuable and worthy of honor because they are part of God's creation. Therefore, we should strive to appreciate and care for our bodies as a reflection of God's handiwork.

2. Inner Beauty: The Bible emphasizes the importance of inner beauty, character, and a heart transformed by God's love. 1 Samuel 16:7 says, "The Lord does not look at the things people look at. People look at the outward appearance, but the Lord looks at the heart." This reminds us that our true worth lies in our character and relationship with God, rather than solely on external appearance.

3. Avoiding Comparison: The Bible discourages comparing ourselves to others. Galatians 6:4 states, "Each one should test their own actions. Then they can take pride in themselves alone, without comparing themselves to someone else." This encourages us to focus on our own journey and growth, rather than being consumed by comparison, which can lead to discontentment and negative body image.

4. Honoring Our Bodies: The Bible teaches that our bodies are temples of the Holy Spirit (1 Corinthians 6:19-20). As stewards of our bodies, we are called to treat them with respect, care, and moderation. This includes practices that promote physical health, self-care, and avoiding harmful behaviors.

5. Love and Acceptance: The Bible encourages us to love and accept ourselves and others as God loves and accepts us. Jesus teaches the importance of loving our neighbors as ourselves (Mark 12:31). This includes extending love, kindness, and acceptance to ourselves, recognizing that we are created in God's image.

While the Bible does not directly address body image, its teachings provide a foundation for understanding our bodies, valuing inner beauty, avoiding comparison, honoring our bodies as temples, and cultivating love and acceptance. These principles can guide us in developing a healthy and balanced perspective on body image, recognizing the inherent worth and value that we possess as children of God.

Poets Corner

In a world where beauty norms dictate the trend,
Let's rise above and find worth from within.
For you are a masterpiece, beautifully designed,
Unique and precious, one of a kind.

In the mirror's reflection, what do you see?
Look deeper, my friend, beyond what can be.
Your body tells a story, a journey so true,
Every scar and curve, a testament to you.

Embrace the flaws, for they make you real,
Each imperfection, a part of your appeal.
Your worth is not measured by a number or size,
But by the love that shines through your eyes.

You are more than appearances, my dear,
A soul with purpose, strength, and endless cheer.
Your heart radiates with kindness and grace,
A beacon of light, lighting up every space.

Let go of comparison, let go of the strife,
Embrace self-acceptance, and embrace your life.
For you are deserving of love and respect,
A treasure to cherish, never to neglect.

In the depths of your being, find self-love's flame,
Let it burn bright, erasing all shame.

You are worthy, my friend, just as you are,
A constellation of beauty, a shining star.

So rise above the doubts, let them fade away,
Embrace your uniqueness, let your spirit sway.
For in this vast universe, you have a place,
A vital presence, leaving your unique trace.

Embrace your body, your mind, and your soul,
For you are a masterpiece, perfectly whole.
Believe in your worth, let your confidence soar,
You are loved, cherished, forevermore.

Remember, dear one, you are truly divine,
With a radiant spirit that will always shine.
Embrace your worth, for it knows no end,
You are loved, my friend, beyond what you
comprehend.

God Bless You

Phoenix Bloom